Anti-Aging Secrets to Longevity and Beauty

The Best Guide to Perfect Health, Healthy Skin, and Happiness

Norah Michaels

Introduction

I want to thank and congratulate you for purchasing the book, *Anti-Aging Secrets to Longevity and Beauty: The Best Guide to Perfect Health, Healthy Skin, and Happiness.*

This book contains proven steps and strategies on how to slow down and, in some cases, even reverse the signs of aging using inexpensive and common household products along with simple lifestyle routines that anyone can use to make their lives more enjoyable.

In a society where looks and functionality are becoming a necessity, more people look for the proverbial fountain of youth in the hopes of extending life expectancy, quality of life, and overall well-being. This book will provide you with tips and suggestions in easy to understand terms with simple to follow suggestions.

Why spend thousands of dollars on beauty products that provide little to no results when all you really need to do is use items that you would normally find already in your home or available inexpensively at your local grocery or drug store?

The billion dollar beauty industry stays in business by selling man-made chemicals that rarely live up to their promises and sometimes results in damaged skin. Natural alternatives have always been the best option when it comes to your health and beauty. Some alternatives are so simple you will wonder why you have never heard of them before. The simple reason? Because no one can make money from something that nature provides for free.

Thanks again for purchasing this book and I hope you enjoy it!

Chapter 1:
Perfect Health

Perfect health relates to overall health: Beauty from the inside out. What we eat and drink shows up in our overall health and beauty and also in how our mood and emotions are affected. Healthy bodies lead to long, rich lives full of energy and peacefulness for a better quality of life. It is therefore important to look at all aspects of what it takes to become healthy inside and out and how to maintain that health for our future.

The Importance of Sleep

We all sleep. Our bodies require it not only so we can think clearly, but so that the body can heal. Without good quality sleep, your cells would not be able to repair themselves and your body would not be able to heal. Sleep is as important as any medication or medical treatment, yet many people do not get enough or do not get quality sleep. Even if you do get the recommended six to eight hours each night, if the quality of your sleep is suffering, then so is the rest of your body. If you feel tired, you're going to look tired, which means you're going to look older than you need to.

Many factors affect sleeping habits: bad diet choices, medications, hormone changes, room temperature, the bed, bedding materials, lights, noises, pets, stress levels, health issues, being overweight, exercise routines, and any number of other factors. There is no one cure all for what keeps people awake at night or what can guarantee a full night's sleep.

Here are a few things that might surprise you that could be affecting your sleep and can be easily fixed:

- **Cluttered bedrooms**: Bedrooms that have too much clutter can cause stress by reminding you of unfinished chores, and this reminder can make it harder to fall asleep or remain asleep.

- **Hot shower or bath**: Taking a hot shower or bath within an hour of bedtime raises your core body temperature and makes it harder to fall asleep. It also helps to keep your bedroom cooler than the rest of your home.

- **The wrong bedtime snacks:** Too much of the wrong foods at bedtime can lead to stomach discomfort or heartburn, nightmares, night sweats, or frequent bathroom trips. Avoid foods high in salt, sugar, and fats. Whole grain carbs, calcium, and magnesium-rich foods can have a calming effect and actually help you get to sleep.

- **Nightlights**: That little light can actually signal your brain that it's time to wake up. Try to not have any light in your bedroom and use the lowest light possible in your bathroom if you do make that middle-of-the-night bathroom trip.

- **Watching TV in bed**: Watching TV, especially if you fall asleep and the television remains on, can have a very negative effect on your sleep and dreams. Television watching can be over stimulating. Try reading instead.

- **Exercising just before bed**: Sure, you feel tired after a good workout but not only is your heart rate elevated, your core body temperature remains elevated for a few hours after you work out. Vigorous exercises are best performed earlier in the day and at least three hours prior to bed time.

- **Alcohol consumption**: Many people falsely believe that alcohol helps you get a good night's sleep. While it may help you fall asleep initially, as the alcohol leaves your system, it sends a signal to your brain to wake up and causes restless sleep from that point on.

- **Pets**: Besides the fact that pets can crowd you out of your own bed, they frequently move and make sounds during the night that can disrupt a peaceful slumber. Some people also have allergies to their extended family members and do not even realize how much it is affecting their breathing. If you must have your pets in your bedroom, the best place for them is on the floor.

- **Medications**: Some over-the-counter medications actually have a stimulant additive to help you keep going during the day. Unfortunately, that means it is harder to fall asleep at night. Check the label on any medications you take regularly and speak with a pharmacist or doctor to see if the medications you are taking are affecting your sleep.

- **Clock watching**: If you watch the minutes tick away and get stressed because you should be sleeping, try turning the clock away so you cannot see the time. The stress you get from worrying about not sleeping will actually keep you awake.

Whatever is causing you to lose sleep, identify it and look for a possible solution. Good quality sleep can take years off your face, improve your overall health, and possibly extend your life. We live in a society that operates on a sleep-deprived schedule that affects finances, relationships, learning abilities, health, and general happiness. Getting good quality sleep in the proper quantity will ensure that you have the energy you need to reach your goals, do the things that matter to you, and spend time with the people that make you happy.

Oil Pulling

Coconut oil can be used for oral hygiene in a process called oil pulling. An Indian medicinal tradition called Ayurvedic medicine from 3,000 years ago taught us how to do this oral therapy by using approximately one tablespoon of oil (usually coconut, sunflower, or sesame) in the mouth and swishing it around for about 20 minutes and then spitting it out (into a trash can). It's called oil pulling because while the oil is in your mouth, you push and pull the oil between your teeth using your tongue to create suction against your lips or cheeks. You can do this for less than 20 minutes, but you get the best results after a 20-minute treatment. (Note: do not swallow the oil or spit it down your drains as it can cause drain clogging issues.) This process helps reduce plaque, gingivitis, the microorganisms that cause bad breath, and it may help fight tooth decay. Coconut oil is the most effective because of an acid it contains that the other oils do not have.

Top benefits of oil pulling:

- Teeth whitening
- Promotes oral hygiene and eliminates bad breath
- Keeps the skin clear
- Detoxes the body
- Improves digestion
- Weight loss
- Promotes normal sleep patterns
- Reduces headaches
- Helps kidney and liver function
- Increases energy

Detox

Beauty detox can also provide benefits for the skin as well as the body and make you feel and look years younger. By detoxing your skin, blood, and cells, your body can function optimally.

To get the best results, its recommended that you eliminate the foods from your diet that are known to cause aging, such as processed foods, refined sugars, artificial sweeteners, dairy, and gluten products. Then begin to incorporate foods into your diet at least three times a week that have been shown to reduce the signs of aging. In less than a week, you should notice healthier skin as well as changes in your hair and overall appearance. The following is a short list of items to try:

- Incorporating foods high in vitamins A, B, and E. For instance, purple cabbage can help lower cortisol levels, which will result in diminished fine lines and prevent new lines from forming. High cortisol levels cause wrinkles to appear.

- Dried seaweed (AKA Dulse) is loaded with vitamin B and helps keep your fluids balanced by leveling your electrolytes. Because it tastes salty without the sodium, it makes a great salt substitute.

- Citrus fruit, all of which are high in vitamin C, can help with the battle against cellulite. They help repair your skin's collagen and make cellulite less visible. It's best to eat these fruits first thing in the day on an empty stomach for the best results.

- Watercress, which is high in iron, calcium, and iodine, helps improve blood flow and allows for more oxygen to be carried to the tissues of your body. This can improve issues with complexion, dark skin patches, and hair loss.

- Beets, which are high in iron and antioxidants, are a natural colon cleaner. Because they help clean the blood and lymphatic system, they increase the blood's ability to carry oxygen, which leads to healthier eyes and complexion.

- Parsley and cilantro both have properties that help your body eliminate heavy metals from your system. Heavy metals can increase cellulite.

- Sunflower seeds are very high in vitamin E, which can help reduce age spots and stop new spots from forming.

- Walnuts are loaded with omega-3 oils, which make your skin more supple and resilient and can help strengthen your cells against oxidative damage. Omega-3 oils may also work to fight age spots, thinning hair, and sagging skin, which all do nothing for a youthful appearance.

Fasting

Another trend that is gaining popularity is fasting diets. Unlike traditional fasting where entire days are spent without eating, the new approach is to limit calorie intake for two days a week and eat normally for the remaining five days. This plan, called the 5:2 diet, or fast diet, stresses the importance of eating high-quality foods on the days that your calories are being limited so that you benefit when you are not limiting yourself. Of course the program works even better if you incorporate an exercise routine and maintain a healthy eating pattern even when you're not counting calories. There are many versions of fasting, and a person should never attempt to go without food if they are pregnant or have other health conditions unless they have the direct supervision of a medical professional. With this version of a fast, on two non-consecutive days you would limit your calorie intake to 500 calories for women or 600 calories for men. Those calories need to come from high-quality food choices and be spread throughout the day. Drinking plenty of water is encouraged. On the other five days of the week, while you can eat anything, it's still best to make healthy food choices so you do not cancel out the positive effects achieved on the two days you worked so hard for an improvement. Besides the obvious reason of weight loss, fasting diets improve cholesterol and glucose levels (which can cut the risk of developing diabetes). Fasting helps you lose fat, not just weight. Fasting helps detoxify the body, which decreases the risk of cardiovascular diseases and your risk of cancer. Other benefits that are being studied are: how fasting can improve eczema and psoriasis, improve the immune system, and increase longevity. And as if that wasn't enough, fasting makes you more aware of how you eat, when you eat, what types of food you eat, and how you might react to those foods.

Chapter 2:
Healthy Skin

There are many books and websites devoted to the use of natural beauty products. You can spend hours, if not days, reading up on information and looking for the fountain of youth. In this chapter we will provide you with a few tips and tricks with the realization that each person is unique and will need to find a system that works for them which they can routinely fit into their lifestyle. Because skin is the largest organ of our body, it is important to remember that what we put on our skin goes into our body.

Natural Alternatives

Coconut oil is quickly becoming a popular method of moisturizing the skin which is effective and inexpensive. Organic coconut oil with no additives (virgin and unrefined) is available at many grocery stores. It helps lock in the skin's own moisture and gives a nice glow. Place a small amount on a wash cloth or cotton ball and gently rub on your face or neck.

Baking soda has been used as a natural alternative for years. For an easy homemade recipe try ½ cup of coconut oil mixed with ¼ cup baking soda which makes a wonderful facial and body scrub. This same recipe can be used as toothpaste. You mix the two ingredients together in a container that you can put an air tight lid on and store it for several weeks. Simply apply to your face with a soft cloth or cotton ball and rinse off with warm water. Make sure you avoid your eyes when applying it to your face. If using as toothpaste, dip your brush into the mix or use your finger to apply a small amount to your brushing utensil. Some people state that they add corn starch to it and use it as deodorant. To do this to the recipe above, add a tablespoon of corn starch and enough extra oil to achieve a thick paste. Dab under your arm with a cotton ball. (Warning: this will leave a white residue on your clothing, which will wash out with normal laundry procedures.)

Facials not only make your skin feel and look better, but if done correctly they can help repair past damage. To save the expense of a spa treatment, many homemade recipes are available which are easy and safe to use. A good thing to remember is if you can eat it, it will be okay for your skin. Some things you can eat should be used on your skin with caution such as citrus juices, especially if you have sensitive skin, because citrus fruits contain citric acid which could cause acid burns if used too much. Many homemade recipes that can be found online or in books available in health food stores will use common household items such as strawberries or blueberries (because the fruit acid exfoliates), bananas or avocados (which are great moisturizers), or honey and oatmeal (which make wonderful skin soothers). You should easily be able to find one that will work for you.

Here is a recipe for all skin types that cleans, stimulates, and revitalizes: In a blender place one cup of a peeled, cut apple, one teaspoon almond oil, one teaspoon lime juice, and two tablespoons plain yogurt. Blend ingredients well until you have a smooth watery all-natural cleaner. Use this in place of soap on a soft cloth to wash your face or body. Rinse with warm water. Store leftovers for a few days in an air tight container in your refrigerator.

Store-bought Products

Moisturizers are the key to slowing down the skin aging process. Store-bought brands are normally full of chemicals that are hard to pronounce and can be hard on sensitive skin. Dermatologists suggest that instead of looking for the most expensive products, you should instead look for products that contain hyaluronic acid (which plumps the skin), peptides (helps natural collagen production), and antioxidants (which protect the skin). They also recommend using natural organic oils. If coconut oil is a scent that does not please you, try sunflower or olive oil. Jojoba oil produces results similar to what our bodies produce naturally to keep our skin hydrated. Many hand and body lotions on the market are now more aware of the need to incorporate vitamins into their products. When looking for these lotions, look for labels that list vitamins A, C, and E as well as moisturizers for skin that will be nourished, healed, and healthy looking. Aloe products have been on the market for burns for many years, but they also promote skin health, even for dry, cracked skin.

For a good face scrub made from natural ingredients, oatmeal, honey, and coconut oil have been proven to work very well. Mix one cup of oatmeal with a half cup of honey and a half cup of oil (coconut, almond, or olive oils work best). If the mixture is a little too thick, add a little extra oil. Rub the mixture onto your face and neck for 3–5 minutes and then rinse it off with warm water. The oatmeal provides anti-inflammatory compounds along with antioxidants, the honey has antibacterial properties and promotes healing, and the oil helps to clean and moisturize the skin without increasing the odds of acne.

If you are going to try at home treatments, remember to stick to treatments that are made from natural products to lessen the chance of allergic reactions. After all, you're trying to look your best, not create further damage. Use caution when searching for and using untested home remedies, especially if you have sensitive skin or allergies. Always try new recipes on an area besides your face (such as your wrist or the inside of your elbow) to ensure you will not have a major reaction that might cause you not only pain, but possible embarrassment and potentially damaged facial skin. While true health begins from within, the products we apply to the outside of our body can benefit us while we change our habits to improve our internal health. True beauty is not just skin deep, it is also cellular.

Sun Exposure

Seeing how sun exposure can cause dry skin and wrinkles, it's important to cover up exposed skin with either sunscreen (SPF 30 or higher), clothing that protects against ultra-violet rays, head gear, and even sunglasses if you plan to spend long periods of time outdoors. The lighter your skin, the more important it is to watch how long you get sun exposure each day. Many clothing lines are starting to feature fabrics that protect against the damaging rays of the sun, but simply wearing a long-sleeved shirt and pants or a long skirt can provide ample protection. It doesn't matter which season is it either, the sun still does damage even if the temperatures are cold. At the same time, it is still important to get some sun every day to boost the body's vitamin D levels, which affects mood and feelings of well-being. 15–20 minutes of unprotected sun exposure is adequate for most people to help the body naturally produce the levels of vitamin D that is required by the bones in your body.

Hydration

Since the human body is seventy percent water, it only makes sense that water is an important factor in any beauty routine. However, it's not only important to consume water on a frequent basis, it is also important to evaluate the type of water that you drink, the water you use for cleansing your skin, and the water content in any beauty products you might use.

Hot water tends to irritate skin and can actually dry your skin out making fine lines more noticeable and accentuating any discoloration that may already exist. A natural cleaner you can make at home uses one teaspoon of honey and one teaspoon of almond oil. Mix the two ingredients well and apply with a cotton ball. Leave on your face for 10–15 minutes and then wash off with warm water. Washing your face at night not only removes the dirt and oil that has accumulated during the day, but it also hydrates the skin at a point in the day when you will most likely not be exposing your skin to further damaging environmental particles or sunlight. While sunlight is important for good health, unprotected exposure should be limited to 20 minutes a couple of times a week.

Another means of hydrating your skin is to use coconut oil. The fatty acids in coconut oil make it the perfect antiviral, antifungal, antibacterial moisturizer for most people. It will keep your skin protected from bacteria while providing hydration. It can be used in place of soap by adding a small amount to a slightly dampened washcloth and rubbed gently on the face and neck. After letting it set for a few minutes you can either wipe it off or rinse it off with warm water. For even better results you can then rub a small amount back onto the skin as a stand-alone moisturizer. A side benefit: the smell is wonderful and your skin will glow.

Of course drinking water is still your best form of hydration. The "eight glasses of water per day" guideline is a reference point, although each person has individual needs based on their lifestyle. Many people report that by sticking to a routine of drinking lots of water, their skin looks softer and has fewer wrinkles. This would match what research shows because when water increases blood flow throughout the body, it improves the skin's density and plumpness, which effectively fills in those little lines and wrinkles. By drinking the majority of your water intake in the morning and sipping smaller amounts throughout the rest of the day, you can reduce nighttime bathroom runs while still benefitting from the hydration provided.

Dermatologists also recommend keeping your environment moist as another means of hydrating your skin. Especially in the winter months, air in the home can become dry due to various heating methods. Adding a humidifier onto your furnace or having a stand-alone humidifier unit can help keep your skin hydrated. Putting a towel over your head and placing your head over a bowl of steaming water can provide the same short-term relief. Try adding fragrance to the water for a natural soothing effect.

It's good to remember that not all of our water consumption has to come from a glass of water. Many of the foods available year-round in the produce department of your grocery store have a high percentage of water. Foods such as watermelon, cantaloupe, grapes, lemons, limes, oranges, grapefruits, strawberries, tomatoes, cucumbers, celery, bell peppers, and lettuce all contain water plus provide many other health benefits that can improve your complexion and overall well-being.

Nutritional Needs

We all know the saying, "You are what you eat." While you may not turn into a jelly donut or a bowl of lettuce, the fact is what you eat will have an effect on how you look. I am not saying it's time to toss everything in your cupboards and become a vegan, although there have been many studies that show that type of diet has amazing results for the skin; however, junk food should be eaten in moderation or avoided completely. Take a close look at the ingredient labels of the foods you eat on a regular basis. Most of the foods we purchase that come in boxes, cans, and jars, are so processed and loaded with chemicals that we cannot even pronounce them. It's no wonder we don't feel good or look our best. If you were handed the ingredients individually and asked to eat them as separate items, most of those items couldn't be consumed in that manner. Yet we continually purchase foods of this nature and stock our kitchens with them.

To have healthy skin, bodies, and minds, you have to make healthy food choices. That means the majority of your diet should be natural foods that are unprocessed. The additives in junk food tend to cause inflammation that damages our skin while fruits and vegetables contain antioxidants and vitamins that reduce inflammation.

While we have a wide variety of supplements and vitamins available that can be purchased at many stores, it's still best if you can get these much needed nutritional needs from the foods that you eat. For example, vitamins A, C, and E are all vitamins with antioxidants that help our skin look its best. Carrots, squash, pumpkin, and sweet potatoes are all high in vitamin A. Broccoli, red peppers, kale, lemons, and oranges are all high in Vitamin C. Olives, raw almonds, spinach, and avocados are all high in vitamin E. Papaya is high in both vitamin C and E. Vitamin D is harder to come by in a normal diet, which is why we acquire the majority of our Vitamin D from sun exposure; however, Vitamin D is found in fatty fish like salmon and mackerel, pork ribs, beef liver, eggs, portabella mushrooms, fortified milk, and cereals.

Omega-3 fatty acids, typically found in fish, helps build collagen, which keeps the skin firm and maintains elasticity, reducing those pesky little lines and wrinkles. Eating lean protein also helps the body produce collagen.

Vitamin C has been the subject of much research. Not only has it been noted that rubbing lemon juice on age spots will make them fade, if not completely disappear, but women that have a high intake of vitamin C tend to look much younger than their peers. While citrus fruits and orange juices have always been known to help reduce the symptoms of colds, it is finally beginning to be studied for its anti-aging capabilities and nerve-calming abilities. Because of the antioxidants found in Vitamin C, it has a bonus side effect of reducing the inflammation of acne, lessening acne breakouts, and is beginning to show up in hand and body lotions, facial moisturizers, and other facial cleansing products. Because vitamin C is a water-soluble vitamin, there is no fear of overdosing as the body will simply eliminate what it does not require. For people that cannot get the needed amount in their regular diet, vitamin C tablets are an affordable option and easily obtainable at most food and drug stores. Look for organic Vitamin C or products produced without chemicals.

As with any food choices, portion sizes can also have a large effect on how our body will process the food and how we will feel and look afterwards. If you overeat, it is hard on your system and your body may not be able to extract the available nutrients from the food you have eaten. Proper combinations of food are important to ensure you are getting a variety of minerals and vitamins with each meal or snack. You can have your dessert as long as you have made other healthy choices throughout the day to provide your body with the fuel it needs to stay healthy and active. Being overweight will not only make you feel older, but it can have the undesirable side effect of making you actually look older than you are. By watching your eating habits, making small modifications and improvements, you can change not only your overall health, but you can improve your complexion, the health of your hair and nails, and the strength of your teeth and bones, which will in turn make you feel better about yourself.

Chapter 3: Glowing Beauty

As we have already mentioned, beauty comes from within. Cleansing the body through detox and fasting helps to make one feel and look younger and that beauty shines from the inside out. At the same time, how we view ourselves can have an impact on how our beauty shines forth. Positive emotions and positive environments can go a long ways towards a youthful appearance.

Self-Image and Stress

Have you ever noticed when someone smiles or laughs how it changes their entire facial countenance? Happiness can actually make your skin radiant. You can't buy love in a bottle, but it may be the most super-secret beauty tip of all times. When you feel good, you will look good.

Instead of looking in the mirror and getting depressed about those grey hairs and all those tiny little lines, look past that into the person behind those wonderfully deep eyes with that fabulous smile. Boosting your self-image has a tremendous impact on how your skin will age. Worry can alter hormone levels and actually cause acne, rosacea, and other skin disorders. Research has already proven that stress can cause hair loss, hives, eating disorders, rashes, sleep loss, and it even speeds up the aging process. So it's been proven that your emotions will affect how you look.

If you spend time boosting your own self-image, you are investing in the future of your face. Work on reminding yourself about your positive traits, your skills and abilities, and the wonderful things that make you unique. Learn to laugh at life and let go of stress before it puts another battle line on your face. Search for the things that make you smile often and surround yourself with them. Spend time with people you love that can make you laugh. Hug often, smile more, laugh deeply, and accept yourself for the wonderful person you have developed into. This will add youthfulness back into your life.

No matter how you look at it, stress makes a person of any age look older. Everyone has stress, whether it's over minor issues or major life-altering issues. Fortunately, we also have the means to reduce and sometimes eliminate stress just by being aware that it is a part of our lives. Stress doesn't always require a paid medical professional and high-priced drugs, which only treat the symptoms and seldom provides a cure. What it usually requires is an honest look at what is happening, what you can and cannot change, and how you choose to react to the facts of any situation. Some people are just more talented at this skill than others, but everyone can develop skills to get them through tough times.

It doesn't matter how well off you are or how much you love your life and the people in it, something will come along that causes some form of stress. It's a fact of life that is unavoidable. Your reaction to that stress is what will make the difference to how it affects your health and the aging process. There is no magic pill that will make stress disappear and if there was, I doubt we would ever be able to afford it if the pharmaceutical companies could even keep it in stock. We could be drugged into oblivion, but the stress would still be there lurking around the next corner.

So what do we do about all this vicious stress? We grab it by the horns and wrestle it down to a manageable size by using stress reduction techniques that have worked for hundreds, if not thousands, of years in various cultures. Your parents probably tried teaching you about the first basic technique as a child when they told you to take a deep breath and count to ten before you said something you might regret later on. Surprisingly, that technique actually works because it forces us to slow down, take a deep breath, and gives ourselves a minute to think about what the real issue is. The key is taking the deep breath, which provides extra oxygen to the brain and allows us to think clearer. The process of thinking about counting to ten actually distracts us somewhat from what the original aggravator was so that some of our anger slips away. By the time you get to the number ten, your response is somewhat different then it would have been if you had allowed yourself to explode at number one. Some of your stress has already dissipated. Sometimes it works, sometimes it doesn't, but it always produces a pause that at least allows you to change your mind about the outcome.

Massage

Massage is a wonderful way to alleviate stress. It helps reduce anxiety and tension while relaxing the body. It makes you feel good about yourself. Even small amounts of self-massage to achy tired muscles can go a long way towards making you feel a few years younger. If you cannot afford to get a professional massage, there are many products on the market that can help you achieve a similar result in your own home. Look for products that are easy to use and can be safely stored in areas where you will get the most benefit from them.

Exercise: Mind and Body

All forms of exercise increases blood flow to the skin and gives it a more youthful appearance. That extra blood flow improves the make up of the skin and can actually help to return it to a healthier, younger condition. So not only does it improve the rest of your muscles and tissues, it affects the largest body organ of all: your skin. Remember to speak with your primary care provider before beginning any new or vigorous exercise routines that might impact your health. The idea is to make you healthier—not injured in the process.

Exercise is not always in the form of physical activity. The mind also requires exercise to keep it active, alert, and fully functional. Many people have found that by continuing education in their later years, they feel energized and filled with new purpose. Hobbies that promote concentration and gives you a sense of accomplishment improve your mental facilities as well as your self-esteem. Activities like reading, puzzles, games, or activities that make the brain engage in strategic thinking has been shown to boost a person's mood and thereby makes a person feel younger. If you feel younger, you will act younger and in turn look younger. It's the reverse of the vicious aging cycle and it's easy and fun to do.

Physical exercise is still important to keep our bodies at their optimal performance. Walking is still the easiest and most likely safest exercise routine that everyone can become involved in. Not only does it give your muscles a mild work out, but it gives you the chance to breathe fresh air and enjoy natural sunlight. No one said you had to run a marathon to benefit from exercise. Of course if you're already physically active as a part of your normal routine, then look for ways to mix up your routine so that you do not become bored and tempted to quit.

Various forms of breathing and stretching exercises have wonderful multi-leveled health benefits. By keeping muscles limber, we are much more likely to stay more active on a daily basis. Yoga, qigong, Pilates, and tai chi are a few methods of exercise that bring great results with minimal dangers of over exertion. These exercises can be done any time of the day and will not normally interfere with sleep at night. Join a laughing yoga class, find a gym partner and go work out regularly, or look for opportunities in your local community to join with other people for similar activities.

The biggest excuse is that as a society, we just do not have the time to take care of ourselves like we should. Now is the time to ask yourself: Do you want to be able to take care of yourself or do you want someone else to be responsible for your care? By taking the small amount of time required to practice the art of self-care, you ensure that you will have more years available to live a better quality of life with yourself being the person in charge of your life. No one wants to grow old and feeble. No one wants to give control of their lives over to another person. You don't need to expend every waking minute to diet and exercise issues in your life, but you do need to be aware if you need to make changes and start to change the things you can right now before it's too late. The important thing is to do something that will keep you feeling younger, healthier, more alert, and happier about your life. If you take the steps to care for yourself now, while you can, you will have taken the steps that tell the aging process to slow down because you're not ready to accept defeat yet. Growing old gracefully does not mean accepting the fact that you are aging, it means learning to dance to a new song that you helped orchestrate by the actions you take towards your own body and health.

Meditation

Meditation can be used for both short and long sessions to ease tension and stress. During the day when you're caught in a situation that requires quick attention, a brief two-minute meditation can soothe ruffled nerves enough to give you the strength to continue. Close your eyes and picture yourself anywhere other than where you are currently at. Someplace comfortable and soothing that brings you peace and makes you smile inside (and possibly outside as well). In about two minutes your pulse slows down, your breathing slows down, and you feel more relaxed. When you open your eyes you should be able to refocus on the problem at hand with a lower stress level. Another method is to focus on your breathing pattern. Sit with your hands on your stomach and simply breathe. Think of nothing but your breath going in and out of your body. If your mind wanders, gently bring it back to your breathing. After a few minutes you should feel calmer and ready to return to the issue at hand. If you have the time available, a longer meditation session of a half hour or more would bring even more benefits. You can either focus on your breathing or find an object such as a candle flame to look at while you think of nothing else but the object of your focus. If you have limited time, set an alarm or timer so you don't lose track of time. Not only will you reduce your stress levels, you will also experience other health benefits, such as lower blood pressure, increased energy levels, more creativity, better focusing ability, and a greater sense of peacefulness and well-being. Meditation allows us to calm our minds and find peace in a normally stressful world. Focusing on our breathing patterns either as a part of meditation or separately, allows us to build concentration levels, reduce stress, lower blood pressure, elevate mood, eases depression symptoms, and promotes better sleep. It is so simple and easy to incorporate into a daily routine. Not only that, but it's also inexpensive and safe to practice. Once a pattern is developed you will wonder why you did not start years ago.

Peer Support

Another method of stress reduction gaining popularity in the Western culture is the use of peer support. While we have actually been doing this for years, it has only recently been given a formal name and recognized as a medical treatment—whether done professionally or informally. Basically, it means to get together with someone you have something in common with and spending time with them talking about the issues in your life and doing things that make you feel better about yourself. In other words, have a positive friend that helps you reduce your stress levels. By spending time with people that make you laugh, remind you of your positive features, and keep you active, you will feel better and look younger because you will have reduced your stress. If you find that your circle of friends tend to bring you down, it may be time to find a few new friends to lift you up again. Trained peers can also help you deal with anger issues.

Spirituality

While we often do not think about spirituality as having stress-reducing abilities, any time you feel a connection with a power greater other than yourself, you feel peace and find comfort. It doesn't matter which religion or spiritual connection you have, as long as you feel you can reach out to something or someone that has more control over the stressors of life than you. Even simply reconnecting with nature can provide a calmness that reflects on a persons' face. Spirituality and religion are similar, yet two different things. Spirituality requires you to look within and is very personal and normally very soothing. Religion tends to involve other people and structures and can be more formal and judgmental. Spirituality spans every culture, age, gender, and belief system and can be a great means of achieving reduced stress in your life.

Reconnecting with Nature

Reconnecting with the world in which you live and looking for the positive aspects of your environment helps to relieve stress as well. We sometimes get so caught up in the busy hustle of everyday life, that we forget that beauty surrounds us. Spend a few minutes looking for that beauty every day and focus on it for a break from your stressors.

Chapter 4: Longevity Secrets

In Nago, a community in Okinawa, Japan, the residents tend to live to be over one hundred years old. They eat healthy, exercise regularly, and drink water that is filtered through the coral that surrounds their costal region. The secret is that the coral is loaded with magnesium and calcium, which helps to strengthen their bones and prevent osteoporosis and arthritis. The combination of calcium and magnesium also neutralizes the acidity level in the body caused by stress, nicotine, alcohol, sugar, salt, red meats, fish and dairy products. Because of this reduction in acidity, they also have less illnesses. Because they feel better, they take better care of themselves and are therefore active later in life. They tend to have healthier diets that are complimented by their active, yet peaceful lifestyles, which is the key to promoting longevity. It has only been recently that scientists have started to research the components of the water that this population drinks from birth on and the benefits of the long-term diet and lifestyles of this remarkable group of people.

Acupuncture has grown in popularity in recent years. The prices have become affordable and locations are available in most major cities. For those that are squeamish about needles, there are several methods of self-manipulation methods using fingers instead of needles at key locations on the body in videos on the internet. A method called ST 36, Stomach 36 or Zusanli, is easy to perform on either one or both legs accessing a common pressure point for relief of stomach and digestive problems including pain, nausea, and indigestion. It can strengthen the immune system and help fight and prevent colds and allergies. It is also used to treat problems in the knees and lower legs, and is even used in chronic disease treatments. It is even believed that this simple treatment can improve life longevity. This powerful form of self-care is quick and easy to do at home for yourself and your family. No matter what results you are seeking, the Zusanli pressure point is important for building and maintaining overall health when it is practiced daily.

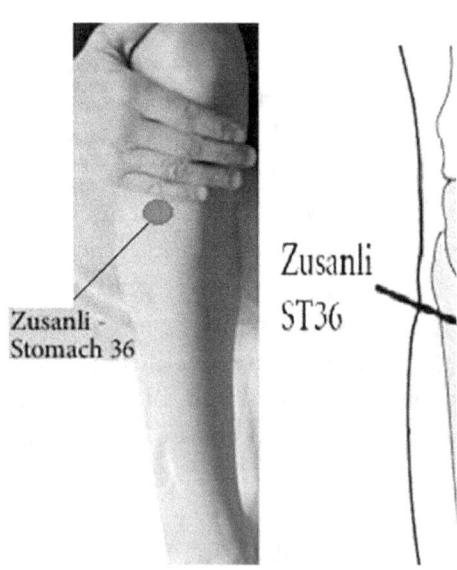

Zusanli -
Stomach 36

Zusanli
ST36

The Zusanli pressure point is located four finger-widths directly below the bottom of the knee cap and one finger width away from the shin bone. Some people will find a slight indentation in the muscle where this pressure point is located. You massage this point daily by pressing on the spot firmly with your thumb and rubbing back and forth for 20 seconds, releasing, and then repeating the process repetitively for about five minutes. This technique first appeared in ancient Chinese medical texts written in 500 AD. In fact, Dr. Shimetaro Hara, who did much research on Zusanli and moxa, daily practiced Zusanli and lived to be over 100 years old.

We all want to look and feel our best every day, and there is virtually nothing standing in our way from achieving that goal. Most of the steps needed to stop, slow, or even begin to reverse the aging process are simple, readily available, affordable (if not free), and easy to implement into our daily lives. The fact is that many of the steps needed have been available our entire life, if only we had been aware of them sooner.

You can take these steps on your own, enlist the help of friends and family, join with a group of others seeking the same thing, or seek professional guidance. The decision is yours to make now that you have the facts to work with and the realization that there is much more information available just a few clicks away on any internet-connected device. So before another day passes, or another wrinkle appears, make the decision to change at least one thing in your life to beat Old Man Time in the endless battle of aging.

Probably the biggest secret for longevity is to be happy with your life, being accepting, having goals to strive for, appreciate everything you have in your life (including people, possessions, where you've been, and where you might still go), finding happiness, and not worrying about every little obstacle that might arise. A peaceful mind and positive thinking goes a long way towards inner and outer beauty. Love yourself; you're the most important investment you have.

So now is a good time to start finding ways to fill your life with laughter, joy, peace, and contentment. The happier you are, the younger you will look. Happiness has a way of healing wounds and fixing health issues. Watch a good comedy or movie that makes you laugh. Surround yourself with people that are happy. The next time you look in a mirror, smile at yourself and see if it doesn't make you look a few years younger.

Conclusion

Thank you again for purchasing this book!

I hope this book was able to help you look at your own beauty routines and find possible solutions to areas that have been bothering you or that you have not had a chance to address in the past.

The next step is to review and revise your current lifestyle activities as they relate to your beauty routines. It could be a simple matter of paying attention to hydration issues or as complex as adding exercise routines into an already hectic lifestyle. Whatever choices you make today will affect the way you feel and look for the future days in your life. Because I know you want the best quality of life possible, I am sure you will seek out additional information about ways to reduce stress, increase happiness and joy, and improve your overall health and well-being. It is my sincere wish that you find and develop healthy patterns for your diet and sleeping habits that will let you live a long and healthy life. I am hoping you will strive to learn more about yoga and meditation practices and the benefits they can provide when practiced regularly as a part of your life. I also hope you will seek to learn more information about natural healthy alternatives for the products you use in your homes and on your body that will help promote ecological awareness for future generations.

Finally, if you enjoyed this book, then I'd like to ask you for a favor. Would you be kind enough to leave a review for this book? It'd be greatly appreciated!

Thank you and good luck!